Distribution, publication, and copying in any form are prohibited and subject to damages.

TEN HYPNOSES

Copying, publishing, and sharing with third parties are only permitted with the written consent of the author. Please observe the notes on copyright and usage.

Distribution, publication, and copying in any form are prohibited and subject to damages.

Copying, publishing, and sharing with third parties are only permitted with the written consent of the author. Please observe the notes on copyright and usage.

Ingo Michael Simon

TEN HYPNOSES

41
RESOLVING BLOCKAGES AND POSITIVE THINKING

Distribution, publication, and copying in any form are prohibited and subject to damages.

© 2024 Ingo Michael Simon
All rights reserved.
Independently published
www.ingosimon.com

Important Notes for Urgent Attention:

The contents of this book are based on the practical experiences of the author with hypnosis applications and psychotherapy in a trance state. Although the author has strived for the utmost care, errors or misunderstandings in the presentation cannot be completely excluded. Therapeutic work with people and the application of hypnosis are solely the responsibility of the hypnotist. It cannot be ruled out that parts of this book may be misunderstood or that the application of a presented procedure may cause an undesirable reaction in the client. The author also assumes no co-responsibility if work with a client is carried out with reference to the statements in this book.

The Author:

Ingo Michael Simon studied psychology and education and is a hypnotherapist with practices in southwestern Germany and Switzerland. With the help of hypnosis-supported psychotherapy, he primarily treats people with persistent psychological conditions. His practice focuses on anxiety disorders, pathological compulsions, and psychosomatic illnesses. His therapeutic offerings mainly include classical and modern hypnosis applications and the dreamland therapy he developed himself.

Copying, publishing, and sharing with third parties are only permitted with the written consent of the author. Please observe the notes on copyright and usage.

Distribution, publication, and copying in any form are prohibited and subject to damages.

INTRODUCTION	6
COPYRIGHT AND USAGE	8
HYPNOSIS 1	10
HYPNOSIS 2	16
HYPNOSIS 3	21
HYPNOSIS 4	26
HYPNOSIS 5	32
HYPNOSIS 6	37
HYPNOSIS 7	41
HYPNOSIS 8	47
HYPNOSIS 9	52
HYPNOSIS 10	55
ALL TITLES IN THE SERIES	60

Copying, publishing, and sharing with third parties are only permitted with the written consent of the author. Please observe the notes on copyright and usage.

Introduction

The series "Ten Hypnoses" is very well known in Germany, Austria, and Switzerland as a collection of texts for therapeutic work and is used by numerous psychotherapeutic practices, doctors, therapists, coaches, and other helping professionals. I am pleased to now be able to offer these texts in other countries as well.

Most therapists have their own methods for inducing and deepening trance as well as for exiting trance. Therefore, I have focused on the main part of the hypnosis. The texts in this book can be integrated as the main part into any hypnosis process. The texts in this collection use various hypnosis techniques. I will not explain these in detail, as I assume that users have the appropriate training. It is also not necessary to understand the exact structure or functioning of the different parts. The texts can simply be read aloud, and they will have their effect.

Decide for yourself which text best suits your client or patient at any given time. You can also combine passages from different texts. It is not about using all ten hypnoses in sequence. It is a selection of possibilities.

I want to emphasize that books cannot replace therapy. Psychotherapy or other therapeutic treatments involve much more. A careful diagnosis is the necessary basis for deciding on the use of methods, including whether hypnosis or one of my texts should be used. Even in this case, preparatory discussions, follow-up discussions during the session, and of course, a therapeutic concept for the sequence of sessions and the content approaches are essential parts of therapy. This cannot and should not be achieved with a collection of texts.

In any case, I wish you much success in your work and I am pleased if my text templates can contribute in a small way.

Ingo Michael Simon

Distribution, publication, and copying in any form are prohibited and subject to damages.

Copyright and Usage

Copying, publishing, and sharing with third parties is prohibited and only permitted with the written consent of the author. Please observe the following copyright and usage guidelines.

This work has been carefully crafted and created to the best of the author's knowledge and personal experience. It comprises text templates and application guidelines for professional hypnosis sessions. The author is a licensed psychotherapist with extensive experience in psychotherapy, coaching, and personal training using hypnotic techniques and methods. Nevertheless, the author and the publisher assume no liability for the accuracy of information, instructions, and advice, nor for any typographical errors. The author and publisher accept no responsibility or liability for the application of these texts and recommendations with clients or patients, nor for any potential consequences or unexpected reactions. It is expressly noted that the application of therapeutic and advisory techniques and formulations lies solely and entirely within the responsibility of the practitioner. This also applies to adherence to the boundaries of legally regulated medical and therapeutic practices. The fact that a book containing action proposals is freely available for sale does not imply that its application with clients or patients is permitted for everyone.

Hypnosis 1

... ... You feel within you the limits and blocks that have held you back ... ... You've sensed that you were no longer free in your thoughts and decisions ... ... that you felt suddenly and repeatedly hindered and restrained ... ... This changed your mood ... ... made you melancholy and dissatisfied ... ... A natural reaction to feeling held back and prevented from moving forward ... ... Now, you've set out on the path to liberation ... ... You have the goal, the firm intention, to free yourself ... ... to break out of entrenched patterns of thinking and routines ... ... to take new paths ... ... and most importantly, to take new paths with ease and joy ... ... Perhaps you want to revisit a path you once successfully walked before ... ... to rekindle a passion or fulfill a need, but today it feels like you can't ... ... What we experience as blocks are often doubts ... ... or we lack belief in ourselves ... ... perhaps because failures or setbacks have worn us down ... ... Maybe this has happened to you ... ... Maybe you've encountered too many obstacles and been held back or interrupted too often, leaving you feeling weary

...... Perhaps you don't even know exactly what it is that holds you back or bothers you ...... It might be a feeling you can't quite grasp ...... But the good news is, you don't need to know ...... It's about finding a way out ...... finding liberation ...... finding the feeling of being free from doubt and fear ...... You need a path that makes you strong and courageous, casting all doubts aside ...... Today, you're walking that path of liberation ...... You're walking that path of liberation now ......

...... Maybe you're wondering how to do this ...... how you can simply let go of the feeling of inner blockages ...... or maybe you've already noticed that for the past few minutes, you've been starting to free yourself ...... You've already taken the first important step towards inner liberation by physically relaxing ...... and with every word you hear, your body moves further along this path into deep relaxation ...... on the path of peace and recovery ...... There's nothing specific you need to do or undertake ...... The words you've heard and the words you're hearing now help you relax even deeper ...... and with the relaxation of your body, it becomes much easier to let go of troubling thought patterns ...... In physical calm and relaxation, it's also easier to release disruptive routines and internal limits … … and to develop new, free thoughts … … You surely know the saying … … "Thoughts are free" … … They really are, because you can now think whatever you want, and no one can stop you … … You are free in your thoughts … … and so you can also think a thought of inner freedom … … you can focus on the thought of liberation from internal limits and chains … …

… You can think … … I am completely free … … and in doing so, reassure yourself that there are no limits within you … … that what you've perceived as a blockage is nothing more than a doubt … … a thought of insecurity … … and even this thought can be replaced with a thought of certainty … … a thought of self-assurance … … with the thought … … I am confident and strong … … This thought now completely replaces any form of doubt … … You think the thought of self-assurance … … You think and you know … … You are truly confident … … You are truly strong … … Nothing and no one can stop you … … nothing and no one can hold you back … … You are free … … truly free … … now … …

...... You feel your body ...... Your body finds more and more peace and relief ...... relaxing deeper and deeper ...... Physical relaxation is a good and very refreshing feeling ... ... a feeling of freedom ...... So now, focus on this feeling ... ... Notice it and enjoy it ...... Enjoy the feeling of physical calm and let your body sink deeper into this quiet and comfortable state ...... Let your body relax deeper and deeper and feel truly free ...... This feeling in your body corresponds with your inner feeling ...... your emotions ... ... your mood ...... the mood of freedom and lightness ...... What could disturb your body's relaxation now? ...... Nothing could stop you from simply enjoying the calm now ...... You can feel the relaxation and enjoy it ...... Just as you can also feel free deep inside and recognize that there are no limits there ...... What has felt like a blockage was nothing more than a temporary doubt ...... a momentary pause that is now ending ...... As your body relaxes, all tensions dissolve, there's no other way ...... and as the tensions dissolve, so do the limits and blockages ...... The blockages in your body dissolve as it relaxes deeper ...... the tensions in your mood dissolve ...... all tensions dissolve ...... all of them ...... You feel the deep calm and the freedom within it ... ... You feel the deep calm that can go even deeper ... ... and with that, you automatically feel the inner freedom, for the two are closely linked ... ... Calm and freedom ... ... Calm and freedom ... ... and in freedom, you feel an opening ... ... a new access to your emotions ... ... a new and free access to all your thoughts and ideas ... ... a new and free access to all your plans and ideas ... ... a new and free access to yourself ... ...

... ... You feel freer in your mood than you did just a few minutes ago ... ... because with the relaxation of your body ... ... with this healing and pleasant feeling, you automatically also feel the liberation from all blockages and limits that may have existed within you ... ... You feel truly free in the depth of relaxation and recognize your own feelings and needs clearly ... ... You may discover feelings you hadn't expected ... ... and perhaps there are even feelings and thoughts you had long forbidden yourself ... ... but now you realize that all thoughts and feelings are always allowed ... ... and your genuine and honest feelings also free you and show you your path ... ... Nothing, absolutely nothing, can stop you ... ... The limits you've experienced as blockages were doubts and, above all, the rejection of feelings you yourself had judged ... ... But there is no judgment for feelings ... ... Feelings are always allowed, just as they are ... ... You allow yourself your feelings ... ... You also allow yourself freedom and openness ... ... You allow yourself to think your thoughts ... ... You allow yourself to feel your feelings ... ... You allow yourself freedom ... ... You allow yourself freedom ... ... Now ... ...

Hypnosis 2

... ... You've often felt uncertain in your decisions and actions ... ... you hesitated and wavered ... ... you were held back by a strange feeling of uncertainty ... ... perhaps by a guilty conscience or the fear of failure ... ... The thoughts of doubt have held you back ... ... more than was good for you ... ... You hesitated more and more frequently, and more strongly ... ... Then, over time, you noticed that you had become less spontaneous ... ... that you had forbidden yourself certain decisions and actions ... ... And suddenly you felt blocked ... ... as if your energy and courage had disappeared ... ... But nothing is truly lost ... ... Everything you once were and everything you could do is still within you ... ... You are still you ... ... with all your possibilities and your potential ... ...

And today is about moving forward again ... ... moving forward in your thoughts ... ... moving forward in your feelings ... ... moving forward in your decisions ... ... and moving forward in your actions ... ... Today, you can already begin to set aside doubts and inhibitions, but above all, you can prepare yourself to move forward even with doubts and inhibitions ... ... because nothing can hold you back if you set yourself up internally today ... ... nothing and no one can hold you back, certainly not what you experience as an inner blockage ... ... Today, you move forward ... ... and in doing so, you realize that you can move toward life, and life also moves toward you ... ... because everything you send out comes back to you ... ... The blockage you've experienced inside has also been experienced as obstacles on the outside, as stagnation or slow progress ... ... Now, you turn back to life, and thus to the outside world, actively, and experience that the attention you give is returned to you ... ... Now listen to the special words of this hypnosis ... ... and let them become your words and your attitude by saying ...

... ... I am ready to look behind the walls of my inner blockages and accept everything I find there ... ... and with this readiness, I have access to the fullness of my emotions and moods, like an open book ... ...

... ... I know that what I experience as an obstacle and blockage is also a part of me that I can accept ... ... and I know that nothing can stand in my way once I accept it, and in my readiness to accept, I already experience liberation ... ...

... ... I look inward, first and foremost, because by doing so I meet myself openly and with sincere interest ... ... for in this way, I come closer to myself and can better accept who and what I really am deep inside ... ...

... ... I take the time of obstacles as a challenge and, despite them, and with them, I face life and my relationships with others ... ... and my fellow human beings also face the challenge of interacting with me, with their own anxieties ... ...

... ... I am ready to step out, especially with the thoughts and moods that hold me inside ... ... and the beauty of life, with all its opportunities and possibilities, comes invitingly toward me ... ...

... ... I end the battle against inner confinement and accept myself with my uniqueness, with respect ... ... and this turns my gaze forward to the freedom in shaping my life, which daily invites me to new experiences ... ...

... ... I am and I remain capable of action and can decide, do, and achieve everything I want ... ... and I experience every day that I am truly freer in my actions than I thought ... ... I move through the day openly, despite my doubts and with my feelings of hesitation, and I allow myself to decide and act against my inhibitions ... ... and in doing so, I find that I can indeed decide and act successfully ... ...

... ... I am a strong personality, and I know that making mistakes is not a shame, and so I walk my path actively and confidently despite any concerns and doubts ... ... and in doing so, I am a role model for others who look up to me ... ...

... ... I am sure that I will become inwardly free, because I move freely and act freely on the outside ... ... for in doing so, I constantly choose to overcome old anxieties and thought patterns that I no longer need ... ...

... ... I am also certain that with my positive and constructive attitude, I recognize every day that I am truly a strong and independent personality ... ... and in the attention, recognition, and respect I receive, I experience the confirmation of my path ... ...

... ... I am unique, and therefore I experience the unique liberation from troubling doubts and thoughts, and I feel truly free ... ... and I discover freedom and independence every day in the opportunities and possibilities of life ... ...

Hypnosis 3

... ... Today, you find a new path ... a path of inner liberation and new perspectives ... ... and for this, you enter a deep inner calm ... ...

... ... Today, you find a new path ... a path of inner liberation and new perspectives ... ... and for this, you welcome relaxation and serenity ... ...

... ... Today, you find a new path ... a path of inner liberation and new perspectives ... ... and for this, you open yourself to the words of release and discovery ... ...

... ... Today, you find a new path ... a path of inner liberation and new perspectives ... ... and for this, you willingly accept all suggestions of the new and the free ... ...

... ... Now, you simply let go of all thoughts ... and clear the way for new and constructive ideas ... ... and you feel that the old thought patterns have served their time ... ...

… … Now, you simply let go of all thoughts … and clear the way for new and constructive ideas … … … and you prepare to let go of old judgments as well … …

… … Now, you simply let go of all thoughts … and clear the way for new and constructive ideas … … … and you open yourself to a completely new perspective … …

… … Now, you simply let go of all thoughts … and clear the way for new and constructive ideas … … … and your gaze turns to new ideas and plans that you now allow … …

… … Open and free, you turn to your ideas and plans … … Now … …

… … Inside and out, you willingly allow changes in your actions … … and your body signals with its calm that you are letting go deeply … …

… … Inside and out, you willingly allow changes in your actions … … and the calm of your body signals that you are now ready to embark … …

… … Inside and out, you willingly allow changes in your actions … … and the relaxation of your body reflects your inner serenity … …

… … Inside and out, you willingly allow changes in your actions … … and with this attitude, all the tensions in your body now dissolve … …

… … Open and free, you turn to your ideas and plans … … Now … …

… … You are now filled with a deep sense of inner freedom … … and this freedom allows you to walk your path with self-determination and engagement … …

… … You are now filled with a deep sense of inner freedom … … and this freedom lifts all limits and doubts within you once and for all … …

… … You are now filled with a deep sense of inner freedom … … and this freedom frees you from all concerns and worries … …

… … You are now filled with a deep sense of inner freedom … … and this freedom invites you to view your path anew and differently and to embrace it … …

… … Open and free, you turn to your ideas and plans … … Now … …

… … Now, you give yourself the official permission … to act only according to your own feelings … … … because in your own feelings, there are no blockages … …

… … Now, you give yourself the official permission … to act only according to your own feelings … … … because only judgments about your feelings could hold you back … …

… … Now, you give yourself the official permission … to act only according to your own feelings … … … because you stand by your needs and desires … …

… … Now, you give yourself the official permission … to act only according to your own feelings … … … because you are the most important person in your life … …

… … Open and free, you turn to your ideas and plans … … Now … …

… … Now, recognize that deep inside, there can be no blockages or limits … … because you can and may decide for yourself what is good for you and what you want … …

… … Now, recognize that deep inside, there can be no blockages or limits … … because you are always free in your thoughts and feelings … …

… … Now, recognize that deep inside, there can be no blockages or limits … … and realize that you can walk any path you choose … …

… … Walk your path … … Walk the path of your feelings … … That is allowed … … That is right … … That is good for you, and most importantly … … You allow yourself to do so … …

Hypnosis 4

... ... For some time now, you've had the feeling of being blocked inside ... ... The same thoughts trap you over and over again, and every time you try to look forward and think positively, it's as if something suddenly holds you back ... ... You don't know why this is ... ... You've probably thought about it a lot and tried to get out ... ... to be free inside again ... ... But somehow, these restraining thoughts and feelings have caught up with you again ... ... You've felt trapped ... ... But you have a firm goal to change this ... ... You want to end the inner confinement and above all ... ... You want to be free again ... ... You want to look forward and see light ... ... You want to feel openness and freedom within yourself ... ... Openness and freedom for new paths ... ... Openness and freedom for new thoughts ... ... Openness and freedom for the new things around you ... ... free from the thoughts and patterns of the past ... ... You can actually achieve this freedom ... ... Today, you're taking a big step toward this freedom that you need ... ... perhaps you're even taking the decisive step, and with this trance, you're already shedding the inner chains and finding an unexpected and immeasurable new freedom ... ... Freedom within yourself ... ... And this is truly possible with this hypnosis because you can experience something special now ... ...

... ... You've probably already noticed that you don't just feel mentally and emotionally blocked ... ... Your body reacts to this too ... ... The human body always reacts to thoughts and moods ... ... This happens to everyone, so it happens to you too ... ... Perhaps you've noticed tension in your body ... ... Maybe digestive problems or headaches ... ... or a greater susceptibility to colds or infections ... ... Perhaps you haven't yet noticed that your body is mirroring your inner blockages ... ... or you've noticed the tension and stress, but haven't connected them with the inner blockage ... ... But today, it's important to recognize this connection, and if you already know it, to focus on it ... ... because body, thoughts, and feelings are always directly connected ... ... and not only do thoughts and feelings influence and change our body ... ... it's exactly the same the other way around ... ... Everything physical affects our thoughts and feelings ... ... and that's a good thing ... ... That's very good, and today, we're using it for your liberation ... ... to eliminate your blockages ... ... and you don't even need to know exactly what blocked you or why the blockage was there ... ... You can simply eliminate it ... ... The benefit of the connection between body, thoughts, and feelings is that your body shows you there are inner blockages ... ... and then it's also very good that by changing your physical feelings, you can also change the inner blockages ... ... You can dissolve them ... ... You only need to recognize that every inner blockage, even the smallest piece of it, can also be found as a blockage in your body ... ... as pain ... ... as pressure ... ... as a hardening ... ... and sometimes as a tiny tension in a single cell ... ... and as soon as you release these tensions, the inner tensions are also released ... ... the blockages in thoughts and feelings dissolve, and you become free ... ... So focus on your body ... ... You don't need to feel the tension now ... ... It's much easier to free yourself ... ... Even if all you feel now is calm and relaxation, the tension is still there ... ... Imagine them as small ice crystals scattered throughout your body ... ... small ice crystals in your body, and each ice crystal represents something that holds and blocks you ... ... a burden that lies in your thoughts and feelings and also shows up in your body ... ... There are many of these ice crystals in your body ... ... very many ... ... Maybe you feel a bit cold as you imagine this because your body is signaling that it's full of the ice crystals of your blockages ... ... That's completely fine and will pass soon ... ... If you feel cool as you think about the ice crystals of blockages and imagine them, let it happen and enjoy the fact that you feel this direct feedback from your body ... ...

... ... And now, imagine how your breath, with each inhalation, flows first into your lungs and from there into your heart ... ... Imagine it, because your body reacts to this too ... ... It responds with a positive and warming feeling ... ... because your heart, the source of your inner warmth, warms your breath ... ... Perhaps you even feel a slight change between cool and warm now ... ... the play between the warmth of the heart and the cold of the blockages ... ... If you feel it this way, let it happen because it shows you that you're on exactly the right inner path ... ... Now, continue to imagine yourself breathing into your heart ... ... and from there, your breath flows into your entire body ... ... like a warm and warming wind ... ... With each breath, you follow this inner path ... ... follow the path to your heart and from there into your whole body ... ... and a warm feeling flows with your warming breath through your entire body, finally reaching every last corner ... ... and the warmth that comes from your heart gradually melts away the ice crystals ... ...

... Picture it and let an image form before your mind's eye, because your body cannot help but react to it and release the tension ... ... and as the tension dissolves, so do the pressing thoughts and feelings ... ... They leave your body, which becomes free ... ... You naturally feel the relief and relaxation of your body ... ... and with it, the relief and relaxation within you ... ... All blockages melt like tiny ice crystals dissolved by the flowing warmth of your heart ... ... Warmth flows from your heart through your entire body and dissolves even the smallest tension ... ... and all troubling thoughts and all pressing feelings dissolve ... ... The warmth of your heart frees you now ... ... The warmth of your heart frees you ... ... now ... ... {approx. 10-15 seconds pause} ... ...

... ... That feels good ... ... You feel the relaxation ... ... You feel the calm of your body, which is your inner calm ... ... You feel the liberation of your body, which is your inner liberation ... ... The warmth of your heart frees you now, and you feel this new inner freedom and openness now and more clearly with each day ... ... because your liberation continues again and again ... ... Your liberation continues ... ... The warmth of your heart frees you today and every day to come ... ...

Hypnosis 5

… … You feel an inner wall, a barrier … … you've felt blocked and trapped for some time now … … by thoughts that you haven't been able to let go of … … by feelings and moods that have imposed themselves on you … … and you've been fighting against them … … because you want to be free again … … You want to be free and enjoy your life … … You want to start your day with a good feeling and enter the day openly and freely … … and experience new things without obstacles and doubts … … That is your goal … … to be free … … free in your thoughts … … free in your feelings … … and then free in your decisions and actions … … And this trance accompanies you on this path to freedom … …

… … You've probably noticed that in everyday life, we often communicate through visual comparisons … … We speak of "icy coldness" when we encounter someone who shows little emotion, or we say that we "see light at the end of the tunnel" when we have hope that the situation will change in our favor … … there are many phrases and expressions that work with visual images ... ... There's a reason for that ... ... The reason is that deep within our emotions, we understand and process images and visualizations much better than words ... ... Words are just the tool to help us imagine such images ... ... to bring visualizations to life ... ... The term itself says it ... ... When we say we "visualize" something, we're talking about imagining something as vividly and realistically as possible ... ... like in a very real and emotional dream ... ... and such a visualization also helps you to release the inner brake ... ... to dissolve disturbing thoughts or thought patterns ... ... You may know what holds you back inside or stops you ... ... what bothers you and which thoughts and feelings you haven't been able to turn off, but definitely want to ... ... Maybe it's not so tangible, but you notice and feel these blockages within you ... ... You want to end them ... ... You can end them ... ... end them with an image that helps you ... ... It helps because your subconscious understands the image and recognizes the chance for liberation in it ... ... and you can be sure, your subconscious will seize this chance ... ... It goes with you and for you on the path to freedom ... ...

... It dissolves and removes the blockages in thoughts and feelings ... ... for your freedom ... ... for a new and constructive outlook ... ... for a good feeling about life ... ... What could hold you back inside was like a wall ... ... an inner wall that you couldn't easily overcome ... ... but today you can ... ... You're already beginning to take it down ... ...

... ... You are actually already taking it down because you're actively dealing with the blockage ... ... You've chosen a path ... ... the path of trance, of liberating hypnosis ... ... So you're already on this path and can walk it now even more successfully and faster than you might have thought ... ... Imagine this wall for a moment ... ... Imagine a wall so high that you can't see over it ... ... It's so high that all you see is the wall ... ... That's how it felt sometimes ... ... insurmountable ... ... But that's not true ... ... You can overcome any wall ... ... and today you overcome the wall that has blocked you inside for so long ... ... To break free from ingrained thoughts and feelings, we also need courage ... ... because every step forward, no matter how much we desire it, requires deep inner courage ... ... You have that ... ... Maybe you don't see yourself as that courageous ... ... But you face your inner wall ... ... You've recognized and are ready with this hypnosis to acknowledge that you need support to overcome this wall ... ... That takes courage ... ... You've mustered this courage ... ... Imagine it like rain ... ... like rain that suddenly starts and becomes stronger and stronger ... ... Just imagine the wall and a sudden, heavy rain that keeps getting stronger ... ... Let it rain ... ...

... Maybe the rain is like a thousand uncried tears ... ... Let them flow now and let it rain on this wall ... ... And before your mind's eye, see this image of a wall being washed away by the rain as if it were made of sand ... ... It rains and rains, and the wall is washed away ... ... The rain of courage washes away the wall, and it gradually crumbles into wet sand, which falls away ... ... Like a sandcastle in the rain, the wall in you melts away ... ... The rain of courage, the rain of uncried tears, makes the wall crumble like sand ... ... And something special happens ... ... Your courage dissolves all disturbing thoughts and feelings ... ... This really works and is happening right now ... ... It succeeds because you have the strength of courage within you ... ... because you have many strengths within you ... ... because, with the image of the wall in the rain, you can activate your strengths deep inside again ... ... and the wall crumbles to sand and clears your view forward ... ... You look ahead ... ... now ... ... {approx. 20 seconds pause} ...

... ... Behind the wall that has crumbled, a new image emerges ... ... an image of a blooming landscape ... ... This is what you've been looking for ... ... Freedom ... ... This is what you've found ... ... Freedom of thought ... ... Freedom of feelings ... ... Openness to the new ... ... an unobstructed view ... ... and from now on, you can once again move forward without doubt and hesitation ... ... leaving behind everything that no longer belongs to you and that you no longer need ... ... You move forward and feel free ... ... You are truly free ... ... and you remain free ... ... today and tomorrow ... ... and every other day of your life ... ... free ... ... truly free ... ...

Hypnosis 6

... ... The feeling of being blocked and stuck in place is a feeling of imprisonment ... ... You have the firm intention to end this imprisonment and open yourself to freedom ... ...

... ... And as soon as you open yourself to what lies within you and what approaches you ... ... with curiosity and interest, and above all ... ... free from fear ... ... you experience a new sense of inner and outer freedom ... ... because then all boundaries and blockages suddenly fall away ... ... They reveal themselves as illusions ... ... as fear and worry that you end ... ... because you have nothing to fear ... ... because with the opening to your inner self, you rediscover your self-confidence and self-assurance, and above all ... ... because with the opening to your inner self, you reactivate and clearly feel your self-assurance ... ... and with this old and at the same time new self-assurance, you walk your path unimpeded ... ... no more obstacles ... ... no more inhibitions ... ... no more blockages ... ... Freedom ... ... only freedom ... ... Freedom within you ... ... Freedom within you ... ...

… … Perhaps you know that a mindful turn toward yourself leads to a physical and mental calm that feels good, just as it does now … … because you're experiencing such calm right now … … with the trance you've chosen, you've taken a mindful and careful path to yourself and are truly caring for yourself … … This is the best condition to adopt a new attitude of freedom … … because that is best possible in calmness … … In calmness, all doubts and worries become quiet … … in calmness, you always find strength, self-confidence, and self-assurance within yourself … … Now is such a moment of quiet reflection on yourself … … a moment of calm and care … … a moment in which your inner self … … your deep inner self can help you more than at any other time … … now this special moment is possible, in which you can truly experience an opening and liberation … … For this, I give you a very special formula … … a sentence of opening and liberation … … What you must do to experience the liberation from all blockages is just a careful turning towards yourself … …

… … Now, turn towards yourself … … Prepare yourself to speak to yourself … … and thus communicate something special to your subconscious … … It is that your subconscious now ... ... in this moment ... ... in this trance is waiting for a signal ... ... Your subconscious is waiting for a signal from you ... ... for your will and your goal, which it gladly accepts and implements for you ... ... makes a reality for you immediately if it senses that you formulate your goal without doubt and without fear ... ... And now you are without doubt ... ... absolutely open to the helpful ... ... You now hear this goal ... ... You hear it spoken by a confident and strong voice that is just like your own feeling ... ... These words are therefore your words ... ... They are your words and are directed at your subconscious, which accepts them and works for you ... ... You say with a confident voice ... {5-10 seconds pause} ...

... ... I open myself to everything that belongs to me and comes to me, and with all of this, I walk my own path in freedom ... ...

... ... And now let these words sink as your conviction into the depths of your subconscious ... ... Allow your subconscious to deeply anchor the heard words of opening and willingness and follow this opening with you ... ... and feel the inner freedom that is connected with these words ... ... Feel the liberation ... ... Now there are no more limits, for your subconscious frees you and walks your new path with you ... ...

... ... These simple and clear words are your new formula for freedom ... ... They free you more and more, again and again ... ... Whenever you speak, think, or feel these words, all limitations within you dissolve ... ... Doubts and fears disappear ... ... Worries and judgments dissolve into freedom ... ... and you feel only freedom ... ...

... ... I open myself to everything that belongs to me and comes to me, and with all of this, I walk my own path in freedom ... ...

... ... Perhaps you've noticed that your subconscious has already established these words, this formula for a new and free path, as a firm belief ... ... as an opportunity and as a constant possibility ... ... and every day, if you so wish, you can activate this inner freedom even more by starting the day with this formula, saying it consciously and mindfully, to immediately feel that you feel even more liberated ... ... even freer and full of drive and energy ... ... You are truly free ... ...

Hypnosis 7

Instructions for Implementation

The following hypnosis text is designed to be used either as a "regular" hypnosis or as self-hypnosis training. If you want to teach your client with this hypnosis how to effectively practice self-hypnosis at home, then also read the sections {Only for Self-Hypnosis Training}, which you can otherwise leave out and still have a good hypnosis for your practice. A self-hypnosis trigger is a signal that initiates the trance state. With its help, even an inexperienced client can continue to practice self-hypnosis at home. Of course, they can work with "simple" suggestions that they can easily remember and that we should prepare, or even with simple visualizations. Triggered self-hypnosis is a very good tool to give the client a task and to support the therapy. This way, the time between practice sessions doesn't go without therapy, but it continues at home. Completely self-directed self-hypnosis, without a trigger, is also learnable but requires a lot of time and practice. Setting up the trigger is a fairly simple task and, of course, relieves the client, as I don't want to burden them with the training of self-directed self-hypnosis. Despite all the naysayers, I also claim here that it's really no problem to teach a client simple trigger self-hypnosis. It's no more dangerous than meditation, autogenic training, or yoga. People survive that at home without harm. I have seen numerous patients in my practice who not only managed self-hypnosis well but enjoyed it. And if a patient likes to do self-hypnosis, no matter how simple the suggestion in the main section may seem, then it's a very good support for compliance.

+++ End of Instructions +++

... ... Today you can free yourself from blockages in your thoughts, from all thoughts that can slow you down or hold you back ... ... You already feel a pleasant relaxation ... ... and in a few moments, your relaxation will go even deeper ... ... and at the same time, your deep inner self, your subconscious, learns how easy and quick it is to end disturbing thoughts ... ... to end the "what ifs" ... ... to end the hesitation and indecision and to be free ... ... You learn this in this hypnosis ... ... {Only for Self-Hypnosis Training:

… You can even learn to do this hypnosis yourself, because that is also easy …} …

… … You easily go into deeper relaxation, where it's also very easy to let go of disturbing thoughts, even blockages that you can't grasp … … To do this, imagine a red rose on a white background … … a red rose on a white background … … Look at this rose … … Just look at the red rose, because this makes all thoughts fade away, and you come to rest … … That's very easy … … Just imagine the red rose on a white background and wait for the deep calm that arises … … … the deep and liberating calm that spreads within you … … Perhaps you already feel how this calm spreads … … or you're already so calm that you feel completely free … … {Only for Self-Hypnosis Training: … Whenever you close your eyes to find deep and liberating calm and imagine the red rose on the white background, you immediately go into a pleasant and comfortable trance … just like now …} …

… … Today, you want to let go of disturbing thoughts … … and blocking thoughts … … Maybe you have a specific thought that keeps pushing itself on you, and you want to end it … … or you feel blocked and slowed down again and again and can't quite say why or by what … … But you can definitely free yourself and let go of disturbing thoughts and sensations to just feel free ... ... to be free in your thoughts and decisions ... ... to approach new experiences and decisions openly and freely ... ... But first, relax even deeper, then it's even easier to truly be free ... ... Imagine you're walking down ten steps of relaxation into deep freedom ... ... and with each step, you say ... ... I relax deeper once ... ... I relax deeper twice ... ... I relax deeper three times ... ... I relax deeper four times ... ... I relax deeper five times ... ... I relax deeper six times ... ... I relax deeper seven times ... ... I relax deeper eight times ... ... I relax deeper nine times ... ... I relax deeper ten times ... ... and then you are very, very deep in an inner calm ... ... Now ... ... {Only for Self-Hypnosis Training: ... This is exactly how you deepen your trance at home, in your self-hypnosis, simply by mentally walking down steps into deep freedom and counting, just as you heard it here ...} ...

... ... Now, in the pleasant relaxation ... ... in the depth of your thoughts and feelings, you can create a thought of freedom ... ... Now you can create the feeling of true freedom within you, and then every path is open to you ... ... Create the new freedom now by thinking ... ... I find complete freedom today ... ... I find complete freedom twice today ... ... I find complete freedom three times today ... ... I find complete freedom four times today ... ... I find complete freedom five times today ... ... I find complete freedom six times today ... ... I find complete freedom seven times today ... ... I find complete freedom eight times today ... ... I find complete freedom nine times today ... ... I find complete freedom ten times today ... ... And then there are no more limits ... ... You are free ... ... {Only for Self-Hypnosis Training: ... And when you put yourself into trance and have deepened it, you can whisper this suggestion to yourself ... just as you heard it here today, by whispering ten times ... ... I find complete freedom today, while counting ... ... once ... ... twice ... ... and so on until you say ... ... I find complete freedom ten times today ... ... It's that simple, and you can do it yourself ...} ... Now remain in this feeling of freedom ... ... Feel that you are completely free in your thoughts ... ... free and can think what you want ... ... Feel that you have become free in your feelings ... ... Nothing can stop you ... ... because you have granted yourself inner freedom ... ... You have allowed yourself inner freedom ... You are free ... ... You are truly free ... ... {approx. 20 seconds of silence} ...

{Only for Self-Hypnosis Training} ... ... When you do self-hypnosis at home, proceed exactly as you experienced here ... ... It's completely simple and safe ... ... Start with the image of the red rose and imagine it until you feel yourself coming to rest ... ... Then whisper the suggestion to yourself ... ... I relax once, twice, and so on, until you say: I relax ten times ... ... Then free yourself from disturbing thoughts by whispering ten times: I find complete freedom today ... ... Then you may rest, and to wake up, imagine standing in icy rain and then simply say: I wake up again – One – Two – Three ... ... Then you can open your eyes and be awake ... ... It's really that simple ... ... You succeed just as you did here today ... ... You go into trance, free yourself, and wake up again quite easily ... ...

Hypnosis 8

... ... You now allow complete relaxation and calmness of your body ... ... because that is a step towards freeing yourself from inner blockages and obstacles ... ...

... ... At the same time, you also allow calmness in your thoughts and feelings ... ... because that is a step towards freeing yourself from inner blockages and obstacles ... ...

... ... You take the words you hear carefully and attentively ... ... because that is a step towards freeing yourself from inner blockages and obstacles ... ...

... ... And you gladly accept the helping words of liberation ... ... because that is a step towards freeing yourself from inner blockages and obstacles ... ...

... ... You now focus only on your desire to overcome all inner obstacles ... ... and therefore, the perceived obstacles and blockages within you dissolve ... ...

...... You focus entirely on the thought of freedom ...... and therefore, the perceived obstacles and blockages within you dissolve ......

...... You focus entirely on the thought of self-confidence ...... and therefore, the perceived obstacles and blockages within you dissolve ......

...... You know that thoughts could block you and can also free you ...... and therefore, the perceived obstacles and blockages within you dissolve ......

...... You are inwardly free, and you are sure of your freedom ......

...... You feel a deep relaxation of your muscles and your entire body ...... and with that, you feel clearly that you are deeply and completely free inside ......

...... You know that your body always reflects your deep mood ...... and with that, you feel clearly that you are deeply and completely free inside ......

...... You breathe calmly and evenly for an even calmer body feeling ...... and with that, you feel clearly that you are deeply and completely free inside ......

… … You experience and consciously perceive every little relaxation of your body … … and with that, you feel clearly that you are deeply and completely free inside … …

… … You are inwardly free, and you are sure of your freedom … …

… … You now focus on the free feeling of relaxation … … and with that, all disturbing and inhibiting feelings dissolve, and you are free … …

… … You enjoy the feeling of calm and relaxation more and more … … and with that, all disturbing and inhibiting feelings dissolve, and you are free … …

… … You breathe deeply in and out and relax even more deeply … … and with that, all disturbing and inhibiting feelings dissolve, and you are free … …

… … You feel only calm and freedom, calm and freedom … … and with that, all disturbing and inhibiting feelings dissolve, and you are free … …

… … You are inwardly free, and you are sure of your freedom … …

... ... You intend to consciously and deliberately allow yourself to think and act freely every day ... ... because that's how you always take the freedom that belongs to you ... ...

... ... Every day, you also allow yourself to think and act according to your feelings ... ... because that's how you always take the freedom that belongs to you ... ...

... ... You recognize inner judgments and blockages that are not your own thoughts ... ... because that's how you always take the freedom that belongs to you ... ...

... ... You repeatedly make it clear that you can end inhibiting judgments and doubts at any time ... ... because that's how you always take the freedom that belongs to you ... ...

... ... You are inwardly free, and you are sure of your freedom ... ...

... ... You have now heard the helping words of inner freedom ... ... and therefore, the known and unknown blockages in your thoughts have dissolved ... ...

… … You have already made the helping words your own … … and therefore, the known and unknown blockages in your thoughts have dissolved … …

… … The helping words have had their best effect … … and therefore, the known and unknown blockages in your thoughts have dissolved … …

… … You have walked a mindful path of freedom and continue on it … … and therefore, you can now and always recognize and find inner freedom … …

Hypnosis 9

... ... You hear my voice clearly and distinctly, and at the same time, you feel the relaxation of your body, you can move at any time and lie down more comfortably if you wish, and that is so simple because you naturally determine what can and should happen ... ... and with that, you open yourself to new thoughts and new freedom ... ...

... ... You can perceive many things in your surroundings even in trance with your senses quite well, for example, you can feel and assess the temperature on your skin, whether it is cool or warm, and of course, your hearing works very well, and you understand every word precisely ... ... while your gaze turns more and more inward, and all the tensions of your body and your deep inner self dissolve ... ...

... ... You can perceive even more, such as with closed eyes, still capture an impression of the light in the room, because with closed eyes, you still see a slight glow or colored pixels before your eyes ... ... and you feel the air flowing past your nostrils when you breathe, if you focus your attention on your nostrils ... ... And likewise, you already feel that you are becoming more free and open inside, you also feel that you can actually remove blockages and obstacles, and that you can really free yourself from internal limits now ... ...

... ... Every perception you take into focus in trance becomes clear, for example, my voice, and you can, of course, decide what is important for you and what you want to focus on, your experience helps you anyway to be mindful and recognize what is important and what is not, and if you are sure that everything is in order, as it is now, you don't need any special attention but can simply enjoy the calm ... ... and then all blockages and limits in your thoughts and feelings dissolve ... ...

... ... You feel the calmness in your entire body, you can naturally also feel all the processes of the body if you pay attention to them, for example, you can observe and follow your breathing very easily and very precisely, and the next five breaths you can also easily count ... {a breath pause, so that the client starts counting internally and is briefly distracted} ... ... and with each number you count, you free yourself from ingrained thinking and acting, with the counting you become free in your thoughts and free in your feeling ... ...

... ... You feel your body and you feel your surroundings, you can perceive the outer and also the inner, your feelings ... ... and with that, you especially feel the feeling of true freedom and genuine readiness to look forward and move forward, and suddenly you are like unleashed and really free ... ...

... ... Now you don't have to make an effort, and you don't want to make an effort now either, and in this relaxed and comfortable relaxation, you can really rest and feel free ... ... and you are also free in your thoughts and feelings, free from everything that could stop or hinder you, and in your inner freedom, you can finally take your own perspective, walk your own path ... ... You walk your path ... ...

Hypnosis 10

... ... You are searching, and today you find freedom within yourself ... ... You've felt blocked and trapped for a long time ... ... trapped in thoughts and feelings ... ... haven't really been able to escape from the same judgments and self-judgments ... ... perhaps it was feelings of guilt and a bad conscience that blocked you ... ... perhaps exhaustion ... ... or there was another reason for it ... ... But it doesn't matter why it came about and why it felt that way ... ... it is more important to create positive and constructive thoughts that lead you to new freedom ... ... So listen to the following suggestions and recognize the words that sound reliable ... ... These words have the best effect ... ...

... You hear my voice clearly and ... distinctly ...

... You feel the relaxation of your body ...

... Make yourself more comfortable ... if you want ...

... You yourself can determine what is allowed to happen ...

… And you open yourself to new thoughts and new … freedom … …

… Your senses function very well even in trance …

… For example, you can feel … temperature …

… You understand … every word … you hear very clearly …

… And your gaze turns completely … inward …

… And all the tensions of your body and your deep inner self dissolve … …

… Even with closed eyes, you perceive some light …

… And you feel your breath at your nostrils …

… And likewise, you feel that you are … becoming more free … and open inside …

… You also feel that you can … actually remove blockages and obstacles …

… You realize that you can really free yourself from internal limits now … …

... You open yourself to new thoughts and new ... freedom ... ...

... Your gaze turns completely ... inward ...

... All the tensions of your body and your deep inner self ... dissolve ... ...

... You feel that you are inwardly ... becoming more free ... and open ...

... You feel that you can actually remove blockages and obstacles ...

... You realize that you can really free yourself from internal limits now ... ...

... You have clear and ... precise thoughts ...

... You yourself decide what is ... important for you ...

... You know from experience that now only calmness is ... important ...

... And in calmness, all blockages in your thoughts and feelings dissolve ...

... You feel the ... inner calmness now ...

... Now observe your breathing ...

... Count five breaths now ... {pause for one breath} ...

... And ... free yourself ... now from ingrained thinking and acting

... Free yourself in your thoughts and ... in your feelings ... ...

... Feel ... your body and feel your surroundings ...

... Perceive the outer and also the inner ... your feelings ...

... Above all, feel the feeling of ... true freedom ...

... Feel the genuine readiness to look forward and move forward ...

... Feel your ... liberation now ... ...

... In calmness, all blockages in your thoughts and feelings dissolve ...

... You free yourself ... now from ingrained thinking and acting

... You free yourself in your thoughts and ... in your feelings ... ...

... Above all, feel the feeling of ... true freedom ...

... Feel the genuine readiness to look forward and move forward ...

... Feel your ... liberation now ... ...

... Now you don't have to ... make an effort ...

... now you may rest as deeply as you ... want ...

... You may now enjoy calmness and relaxation ...

... and the ... freedom ... of your thoughts and feelings ...

... You may now walk your own path, in ... inside and outside ...

... You may now be yourself, in ... freedom ... ... freedom ... in your thoughts and feelings ...

... You ... walk your path ... ... You are truly ... free ...

All Titles in the Series

Volume 1: Smoking Cessation
Volume 2: Anxiety and Restlessness
Volume 3: Burnout
Volume 4: Reducing Overweight
Volume 5: Coping with the Past
Volume 6: Suicidal Thoughts and Attempts
Volume 7: Psycho-Oncology
Volume 8: Obsessions and Tics
Volume 9: Self-Confidence and Decision-Making
Volume 10: Grief Work
Volume 11: Psychosomatics
Volume 12: Chronic Pain
Volume 13: Depressive Thoughts
Volume 14: Panic Attacks
Volume 15: Domestic Violence, Victim Support
Volume 16: Post-Traumatic Stress
Volume 17: Exam Anxiety and Stage Fright
Volume 18: Anti-Violence Training, Offender Support
Volume 19: Addiction Tendencies
Volume 20: Social Phobia and Fear of Contact
Volume 21: Nail Biting
Volume 22: Self-Awareness and Self-Love
Volume 23: Teeth Grinding and Night Clenching
Volume 24: Feelings of Guilt
Volume 25: Fear in Crowds
Volume 26: Fear of Flying, Aviophobia
Volume 27: Fear in Enclosed Spaces, Claustrophobia
Volume 28: Tinnitus, Ear Noises
Volume 29: Fear of Heights
Volume 30: Neurodermatitis

Volume 31: Finding Inner Balance
Volume 32: Overcoming Loneliness
Volume 33: Fear of Illness, Hypochondria
Volume 34: Anticipatory Anxiety, Fear of Fear
Volume 35: Jealousy in Relationships
Volume 36: Driving Anxiety
Volume 37: New Start after Separation
Volume 38: Fear of Injections
Volume 39: Heart Anxiety Neurosis
Volume 40: Overcoming Resentment and Anger
Volume 41: Resolving Blockages and Positive Thinking
Volume 42: Stress Reduction, Stress Management
Volume 43: Body Relaxation
Volume 44: Deep Relaxation
Volume 45: Fear of the Dark
Volume 46: Falling Asleep and Staying Asleep
Volume 47: Compulsive Buying
Volume 48: Restless Legs Syndrome
Volume 49: Bulimia
Volume 50: Anorexia
Volume 51: Overcoming Nightmares
Volume 52: Imagined Deformity
Volume 53: Overcoming Distrust, Finding Trust
Volume 54: Processing Failures
Volume 55: Humiliation, Emotional Hurt
Volume 56: Distressing Compassion, Vicarious Suffering
Volume 57: Self-Forgiveness
Volume 58: Self-Awareness, Self-Confidence
Volume 59: Saying No
Volume 60: Assertiveness
Volume 61: Setting Boundaries and Self-Assertion
Volume 62: Decision-Making Ability

Volume 63: Success Orientation
Volume 64: Ruminating, Circular Thinking
Volume 65: Accepting Pregnancy
Volume 66: Birth Preparation
Volume 67: Spiritual Opening
Volume 68: Joy of Life and Inner Lightness
Volume 69: Patience and Inner Peace
Volume 70: Fibromyalgia and Rheumatism
Volume 71: Irritable Bowel Syndrome, Crohn's Disease
Volume 72: Fear of Nausea, Emetophobia
Volume 73: Stuttering and Cluttering, Speech Flow Disorders
Volume 74: Concentration and Knowledge Anchoring
Volume 75: Vitality and Spontaneity
Volume 76: Searching for Meaning and Finding Goals
Volume 77: Life Crises, Life Events
Volume 78: Workaholism, Goal Obsession
Volume 79: Helper Syndrome, Helpless Helpers
Volume 80: Medication Abuse
Volume 81: Gambling Addiction
Volume 82: Internet Addiction, Smartphone Addiction
Volume 83: Hoarding Disorder, Compulsive Collecting
Volume 84: Conspiracy Thoughts, Overvalued Ideas
Volume 85: Fear of Operations and Treatments
Volume 86: Fear of Aging
Volume 87: Travel Anxiety
Volume 88: Anxiety When Urinating, Paruresis
Volume 89: Fear of Intimacy and Togetherness
Volume 90: Fear of Blushing
Volume 91: Coming Out in Homosexuality
Volume 92: Charisma Training
Volume 93: Migraines and Chronic Headaches
Volume 94: Overcoming Allergies, Bronchial Asthma

Volume 95: Normalizing Blood Pressure
Volume 96: Compulsive Perfectionism
Volume 97: Sports Hypnosis, Motivation
Volume 98: Sports Hypnosis, Performance Enhancement
Volume 99: Determination and Focus
Volume 100: Encountering the Inner Child
Volume 101: Cravings, Binge Eating
Volume 102: Stimulating Metabolism
Volume 103: Bipolar Mood Swings
Volume 104: Borderline, Identity Crises
Volume 105: Hypomania, Euphoria, Mania
Volume 106: Restlessness, Agitation
Volume 107: Nervous Breakdown
Volume 108: Adjustment Disorders
Volume 109: Self-Alienation, Depersonalization
Volume 110: Ending Self-Pity
Volume 111: Primary Gain of Illness
Volume 112: Secondary Gain of Illness
Volume 113: Bullying, Victim Support
Volume 114: Letting Go of Envy and Jealousy
Volume 115: Fear of Spiders, Arachnophobia
Volume 116: Fear of Dogs or Cats
Volume 117: Fear of Strangers, Xenophobia
Volume 118: Excessive Worries, Generalized Anxiety
Volume 119: Strengthening Sense of Responsibility
Volume 120: Unrequited Love, Heartache
Volume 121: Work-Life Balance
Volume 122: Letting Go of Unattainable Goals
Volume 123: Allowing and Accepting Help
Volume 124: Letting Go of Adult Children
Volume 125: Tourette Syndrome
Volume 126: Life Changes and New Starts

Volume 127: Accepting Life in a Wheelchair
Volume 128: Understanding and Overcoming Homesickness
Volume 129: Understanding and Overcoming Wanderlust
Volume 130: Dizziness, Meniere's Disease
Volume 131: Overcoming Aggression
Volume 132: Cutting and Self-Harm
Volume 133: Hair Pulling, Trichotillomania
Volume 134: Postpartum Depression
Volume 135: For Relatives of Dementia Patients
Volume 136: Self-Harm, Artificial Disorders
Volume 137: Activating Self-Healing Powers
Volume 138: Preventing Depression Relapse
Volume 139: Reactive Psychoses, Follow-Up
Volume 140: Obsessive Thoughts and Impulses
Volume 141: Compulsive Checking
Volume 142: Compulsive Counting, Symmetry Obsession
Volume 143: Compulsive Washing, Cleanliness Obsession
Volume 144: Compulsive Questioning
Volume 145: Dissociative Paralysis
Volume 146: Phantom Pain
Volume 147: Overcoming Complaining
Volume 148: Hay Fever, Pollen Allergy
Volume 149: Sexual Abuse, Victim Support
Volume 150: Standing Strong Against Sexism, #metoo
Volume 151: Binge Eating
Volume 152: Overcoming Thoughts of Revenge
Volume 153: Detachment from the Aggressor, Stockholm Syndrome
Volume 154: Courage to Separate
Volume 155: Chronic Fatigue, Exhaustion
Volume 156: Fear of the Future, Existential Anxiety
Volume 157: Excessive Worry About Children
Volume 158: Fear of Failure

Volume 159: Ending Distrust and Control
Volume 160: Dejection, Dysphoria
Volume 161: Boreout, Chronic Boredom
Volume 162: Bipolar Disorders, Relapse Prevention
Volume 163: Mania, Relapse Prevention
Volume 164: Nihilism, Feelings of Worthlessness
Volume 165: Thumb Sucking
Volume 166: Being Brave
Volume 167: Being Proud
Volume 168: Overcoming Shyness
Volume 169: Being Able to Delegate Responsibility
Volume 170: Being Able to Show Emotions
Volume 171: Letting Go of Guilt, Victim Support
Volume 172: Processing Guilt, Offender Support
Volume 173: Mood Swings, Cyclothymia
Volume 174: Lack of Drive, Vital Sadness
Volume 175: Hearing Voices with Reality Reference
Volume 176: Confident Communication
Volume 177: Standing Up for Oneself
Volume 178: Taking New Paths
Volume 179: Confident Job Application
Volume 180: No Longer Being Taken Advantage Of
Volume 181: End of Submissiveness
Volume 182: Depressive Numbness
Volume 183: Mood Drops, Affective Incontinence
Volume 184: Mood Instability
Volume 185: Somatoform Disorders
Volume 186: Stomach Ulcer, Psychosomatic
Volume 187: Accepting Amputation
Volume 188: Overcoming and Letting Go of Hatred
Volume 189: Ending Accusations
Volume 190: Allowing Tears, Being Able to Cry

Volume 191: Finding and Sorting Repressed Feelings
Volume 192: Somatoform Pain
Volume 193: Living Autonomously
Volume 194: Anhedonia, Joylessness
Volume 195: Persistent Sadness
Volume 196: Obesity, Food Addiction
Volume 197: Parents of Abused Children
Volume 198: Letting Go and Letting Be
Volume 199: Childhood Sexual Abuse
Volume 200: Fear of Loss

www.ingramcontent.com/pod-product-compliance
Lightning Source LLC
Chambersburg PA
CBHW030503220526
45464CB00006B/2632